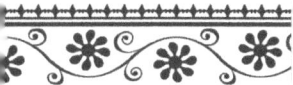

The LaLa Sutras of the dolly alanna™

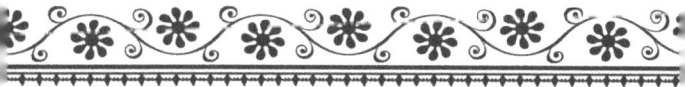

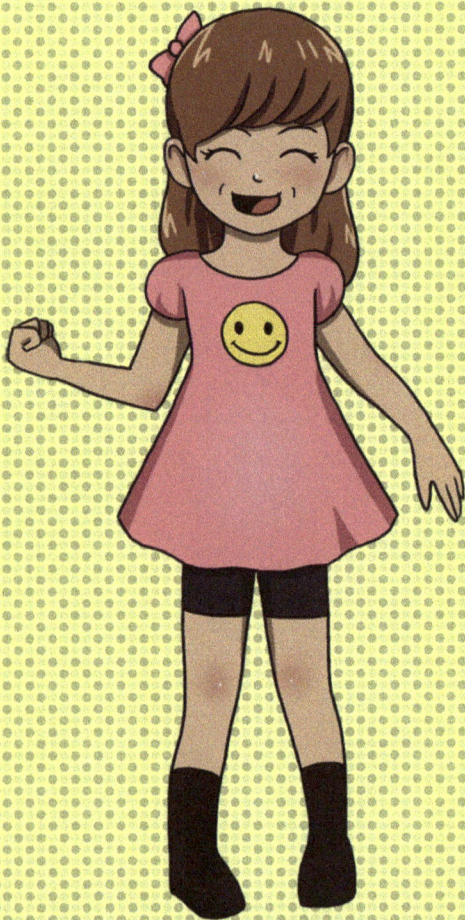

1: i am happy

Each moment I have a choice to be happy.

I AM Happy when I win, and I AM Happy when I see others win. I will not let anything take away my happiness, because the choice to be happy is an endless gift to both myself and others.

No matter what is happening around me I choose to be happy!

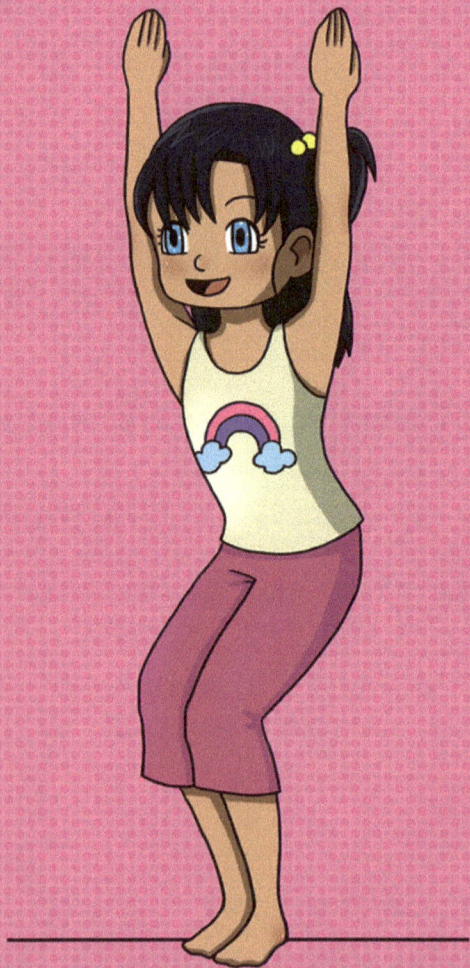

2: i am active

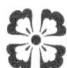

When I AM Active, I feel great! My body and mind need consistent activity to stay healthy and fit.

I AM Active every day, and I love playing fun games and sports with my friends. It's even better when we can play outside in Nature.

I am turning off my computer and TV to go play right now!

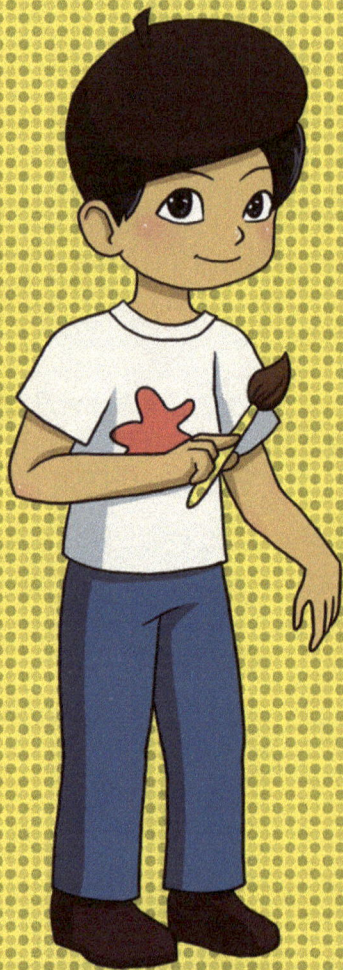

3: i am creative

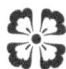

I enjoy creating things that express my feelings, thoughts, dreams, and opinions. Sometimes I color, paint, write stories, sing, dance, design clothes, discover new programs, concepts & theories.

I love mixing and playing with color, even if only black & white.

My creativity shines through best when I listen to how I feel & express myself truthfully through my art.

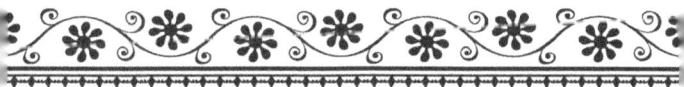

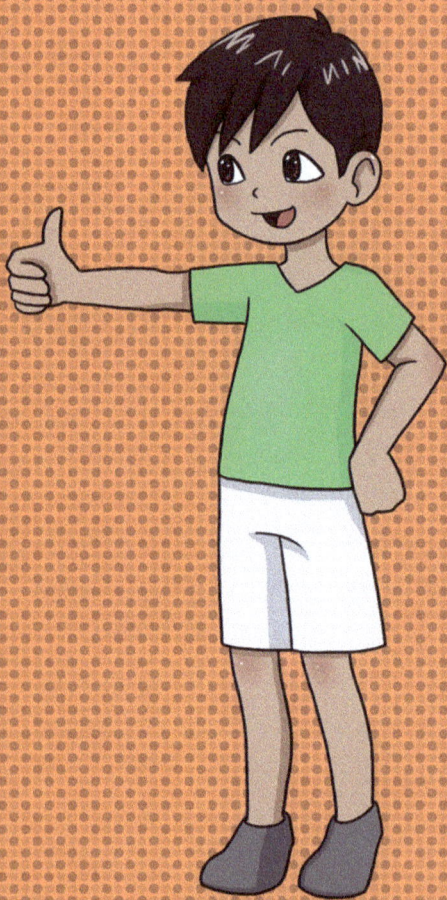

4: i am kind

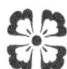

It is important to be kind to all beings, including young and old people, all colors of people, rich and poor, disadvantaged - and to all animals.

Create a way to show kindness to each person you meet. Show your kindness with a compliment, helping with a task, or simply a smile.

When others are not kind to you, calmly walk away. Silently wish them peace and happiness from afar.

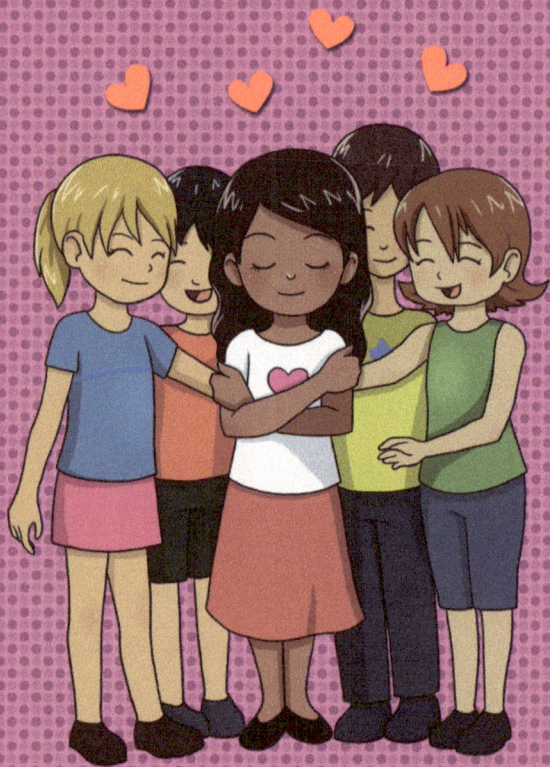

5: i am loved

❀

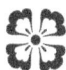

I was born from the energy of love and my soul is the essence of love. I am loved for who I am, unique & true. Knowing that the moments of my life are short, I choose to feel love in all of them.

I, too, love the soul of all beings, no matter what they look like or do.

Regardless of what other people say or how they behave I know that I am unconditionally loved right now.

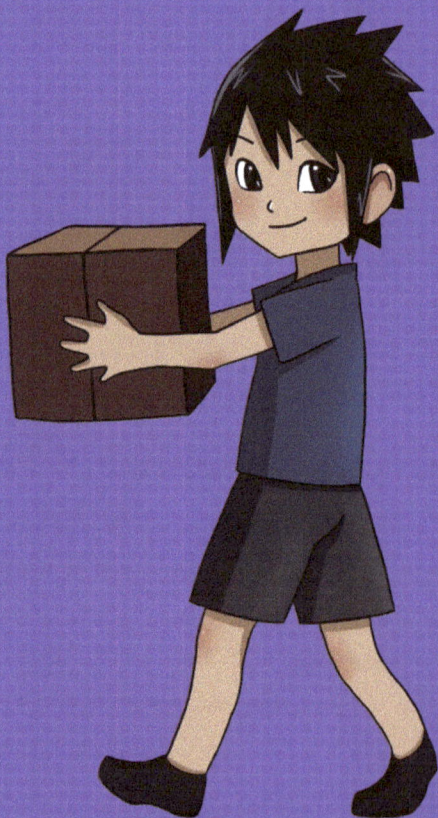

6: i am helpful

❀

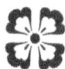

I love working in teams, and I enjoy helping other people whenever I can. I do not expect anything in return for my help. My offer is a sincere and pure gift.

If feels great to help other people, and sometimes I think I may receive more benefit than the person I helped.

Ask yourself how you can be more helpful to your family and friends. You can make any task fun!

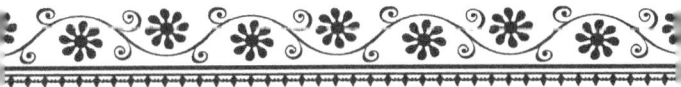

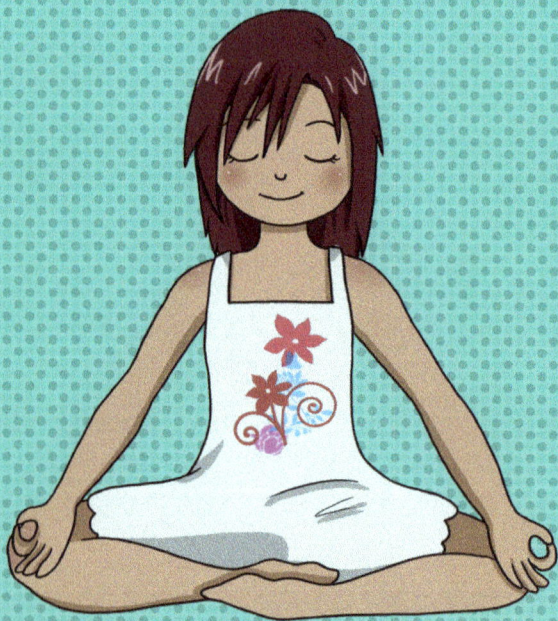

7: i am aware

❀

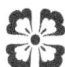

My mind is capable of infinitely great
things that we often do not use. To
develop the power of my mind, I enjoy
meditation and focus. I practice being
aware of what is happening around me.

I enjoy being still, calm, and focused.
This restores my body and it
strengthens my awareness.

Every day I sit quietly for at least
15 minutes while being aware of
how I feel and what I sense.

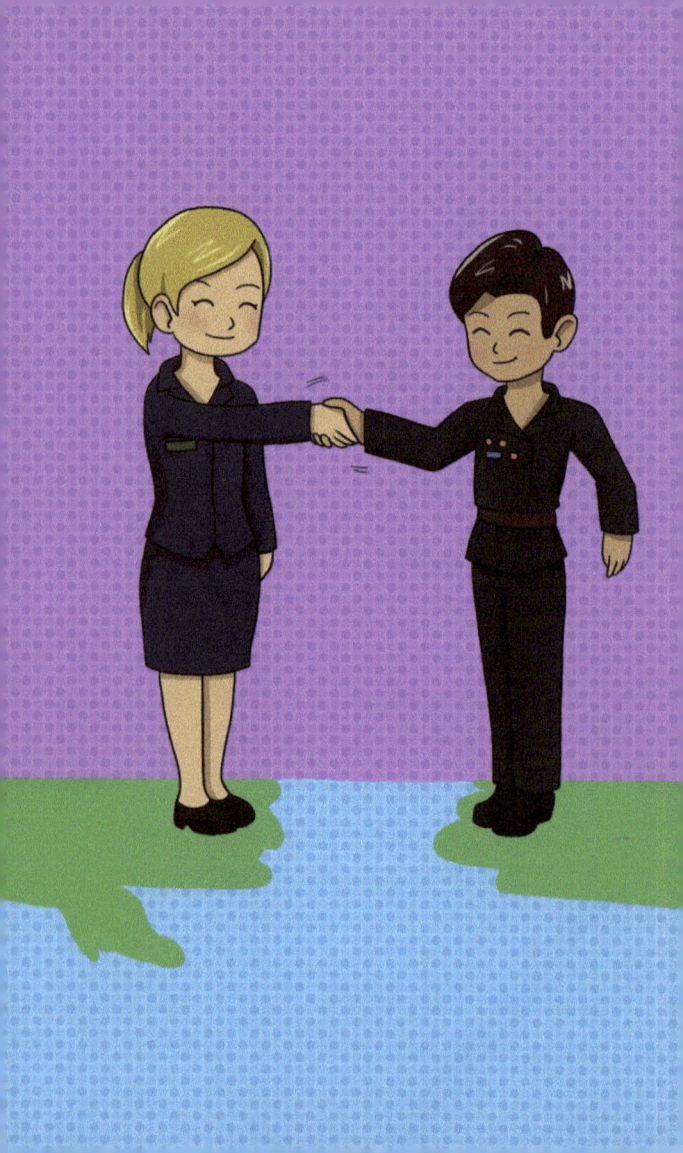

8: i am peaceful

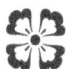

If I have disagreements with others,
I will always strive to seek peaceful
solutions. I strive to express my needs
and opinions without hurting or
insulting others, even if they hurt me.

I will walk away from people or
situations that are hurtful or violent
as it is important to protect myself.

I seek to be fair, kind, and peaceful
to everyone that I meet.
I AM a positive force. I AM Peaceful.

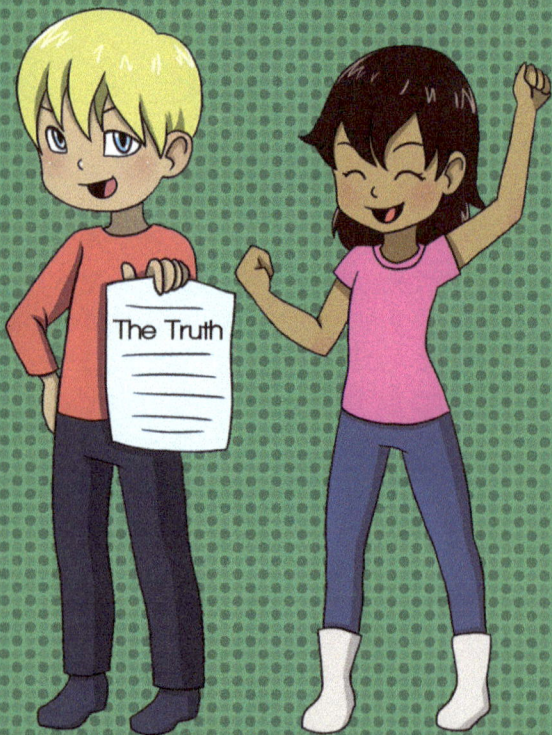

The Truth

9: i am honest

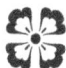

For others to trust me, I AM Honest.
To be honest, all of my words and
actions are true. Living true creates
peace and honor within me.

There is always a way to be honest
without hurting someone else's feelings.
I share how I feel thoughtfully.

By living honestly, I am true to my
promises. I do not cheat nor do
I take anything that is not mine
without permission.

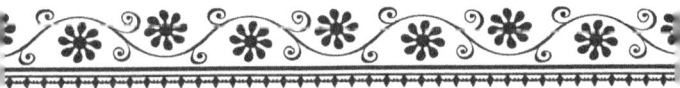

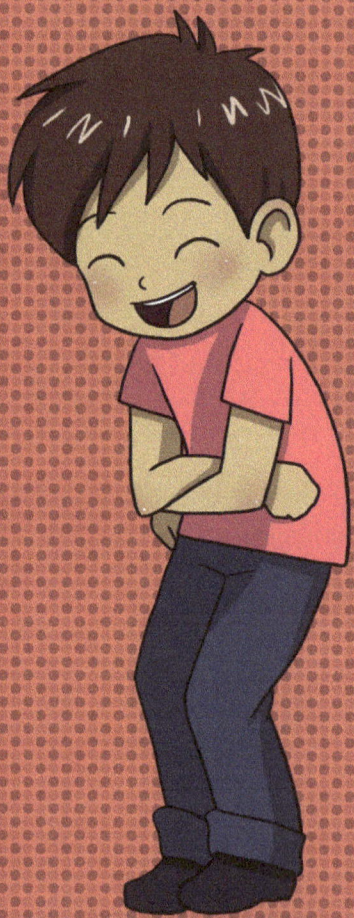

10: i am laughing

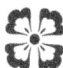

Laughter is a pure expression of Joy.
When I AM Laughing I heal myself
and those around me.

I enjoy people who make me laugh.
I love making other people laugh.
Laughter often lightens a heavy
situation & allows souls to positively
connect, regardless of language.

When I feel tense, angry, or frustrated
I will seek to find humor in the situation.
Laughter truly is the greatest medicine.

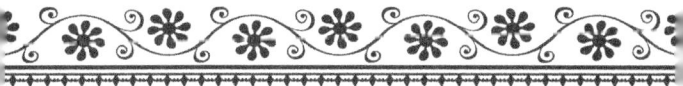

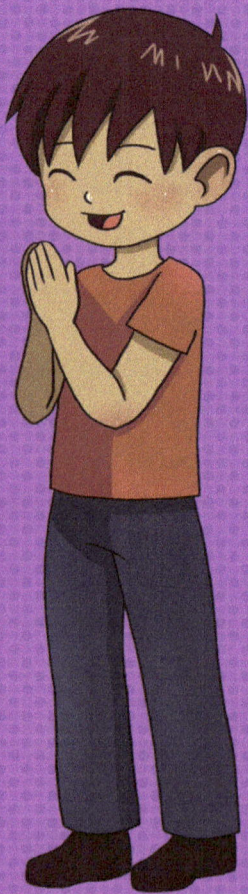

11: i am grateful

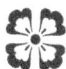

There is so much for me to be grateful for. I AM Grateful to be alive, healthy, loved, and fed. To have a home, family, and friends is a great treasure that many people in the world do not have.

Every day I take time to be thankful for what I have. I wish for all beings to be happy and loved.

May I never take for granted my countless blessings, and always be humble with Gratitude.

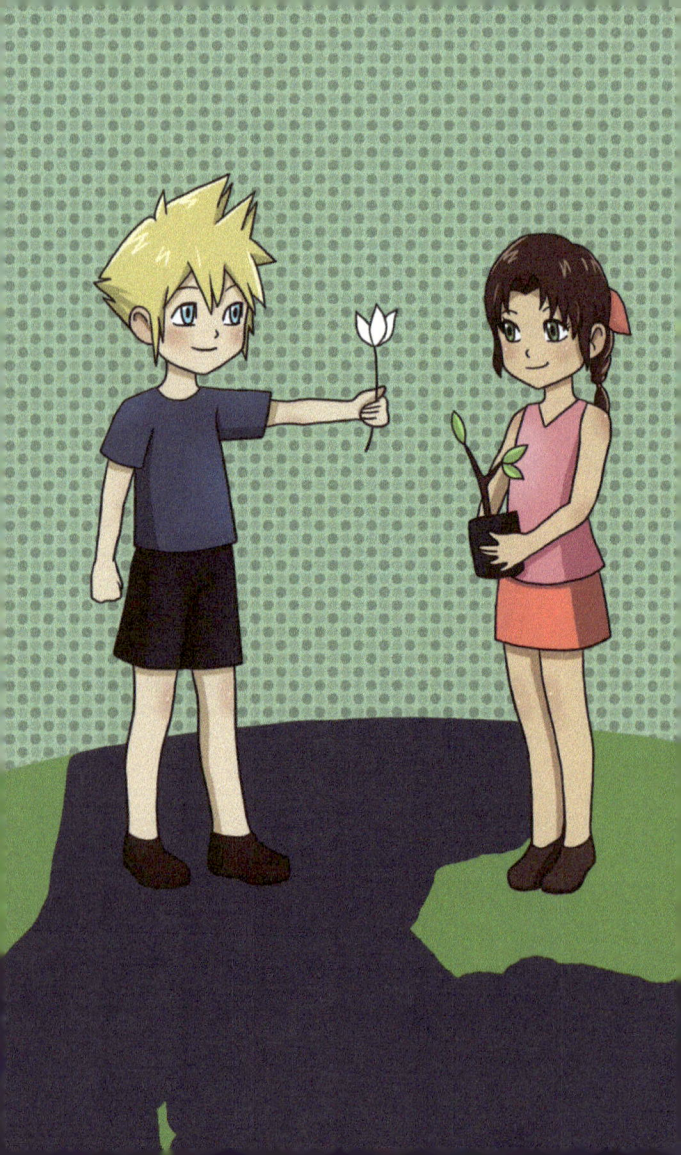

12: i am making the world better

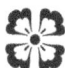

❀

I care about our beautiful planet and I respect Nature in its organic perfection. I AM Making the World Better.

I choose biodegradable products, I do not waste natural resources, I avoid harsh chemicals, and I care for plants and animals with loving kindness.

I am a positive contribution to our world and I am conscious of what I consume and use.

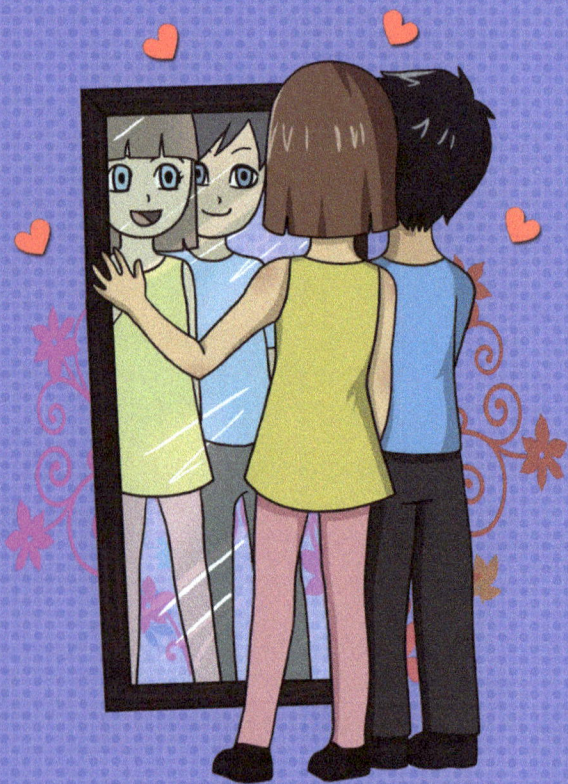

13: i am perfect, as i am.

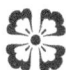

There is no one in the entire Universe exactly like me.

I am in awe of who I am, and I choose to live as my true self. I do not care to look like anyone else to be accepted.

I live my life honoring my spirit. I am unafraid of being judged, rejected, or disliked for being courageously unique and true to myself.

I AM Perfect, exactly as I am.

www.ingramcontent.com/pod-product-compliance
Lightning Source LLC
Chambersburg PA
CBHW052013030426
42334CB00029BA/3210